KETO INGREDIENT COOK BOOK

The Most Simple, Easy, And Effective Guide To Starting A Ketogenic Diet And Lifestyle For Long-Term Health

Margaret Peter

TABLE OF CONTENTS

INTRODUCTION

There is no greater reason to diet than for your personal health and well being. Those people who are overweight know better than most the risks and possible consequences which will result due to our weight. very similar to smokers however, the risks don't always seem quite so cut and dry until we reach our very own turning point. Whether your eating habits are born of an addiction to certain foods, an emotional need, or years of learned behavior and conditioning things won't change until you completely adjust your eating habits and your lifestyle choices.

Dieting for many has become a way of life in and of itself with people rapidly flip-flopping or yo-yoing from one diet to a different with little success and growing despair over a sheer lack of results. the reality is that until you opt to forgive yourself for your failures and obtain right back on the wagon, so to talk , after slump no diet goes to achieve success . an easy diet isn’t getting to magically make the pounds disappear and constantly depriving yourself of these belongings you enjoy most may have a more detrimental effect than a positive effect.

The number one thing most people ought to learn is that dieting isn’t always a good thing. What most people who are overweight need more than anything is to include positive lifestyle changes into their daily routines. People scoff at the notion of taking the stairs or parking farther away and yet those are perfectly plausible methods of working a bit more physical activity into your day. If those don't work for you ways about learning to dance?

Seriously, there are beginner dance classes in most communities which will welcome and invite dances of all ages, sizes, and fitness levels if you're willing to make the effort. What a great way to get fit, learn something new, and celebrate without filling deprived.

Another great point about an activity like a dance class (consider ballroom dance along with your significant other) is that you aren't eating or tempted to eat during the time that you are dancing in most cases. Another great point is that you simply are burning those calories you didn’t eat. If dancing isn’t you thing, try joining a walking club or finding another hobby. Anything that gets you on your feet and faraway from the temptation of your refrigerator may be a good thing when it involves dieting and weight loss. you can't lose a big amount of weight by dieting alone. you want to incorporate fitness into your daily routine so as to achieve those immediate and visually stunning results that a lot of dieters hope to achieve.

Another pitfall when it involves dieting is that people quit far too quickly. just as the results are beginning and progressing people get uninterested in the method or frustrated that they aren't accomplishing enough dramatic weight loss as quickly as they had hoped and give up all together marking off yet one more failure when they could have achieved greater success than ever before if they had cursed with their original diet plan a touch longer.

CHAPTER ONE

What Is A Ketogenic Diet?

The full name is the Ketogenic Diet, because it forces your body into a ketogenic state. The ketogenic diet is a high-fat, low-carb diet originally invented back in the 1920s as a treatment for childhood epilepsy.

If you go on a ketogenic diet, you'll be getting around 80% of your calories from fat, which the body burns as fuel when it can't get carbs.

You'll also be dropping your carb intake to about 5% of total daily calories and getting the rest of the 15-20% from proteins. This is a fairly drastic departure from what we all learned in school as a healthy, well-balanced diet which typically consists of: 20-35% protein, 45-65% carbs, and only 10-35% fat.

While you follow a keto diet, your body will become very good at burning fat, which of course, is exactly what you want when you're trying to lose weight.

It also helps turn your own fat into ketones in your liver, which your brain can use for energy. This diet is known to drastically lower blood sugar and insulin levels, which is where the diabetic benefits come in.

CHAPTER TWO

Types Of Keto Diets

There are two basic types of keto diet: standard and high protein.

The standard diet is the one discussed above, with around 70-80% fat, around 20% protein, and only 5-10% carbs.

The high protein keto diet, just as it sounds, tweaks the proportions to add more proteins.

You drop the fat to around 60% and increase the protein percentage to 35%.

Bodybuilders and athletes often need more carbs for fast energy, so sometimes they'll tweak, and play with that carb percentage.

Some of them will also follow what they call a cyclical keto diet, which follows the standard diet for a certain number of days, followed by a couple of higher-carb days. It's often also called "carb cycling".

Others will just increase the number of carbs they consume right before a workout (a targeted keto diet).

The standard and high-protein diets have been studied far more extensively than the cyclical or targeted diets, so in this special report, we'll be mostly talking about the standard diet.

CHAPTER THREE

Keto Basics

The ketogenic diet is a very low carb, high fat diet that shares many similarities with the Atkins and low carb diets.

It involves drastically reducing carbohydrate intake and replacing it with fat. This reduction in carbs puts your body into a metabolic state called ketosis.

When this happens, your body becomes incredibly efficient at burning fat for energy. It also turns fat into ketones within the liver, which can supply energy for the brain

Ketogenic diets can cause significant reductions in glucose and insulin levels. This, along side the increased ketones, has some health benefits

Different types of ketogenic diets

There are several versions of the ketogenic diet, including:

• Standard ketogenic diet (SKD): this is a really low carb, moderate protein and high fat diet. It typically contains 70% fat, 20% protein, and only 10% carbs

• Cyclical ketogenic diet (CKD): This diet involves periods of upper carb refeeds, like 5 ketogenic days followed by 2 high carb days.

• Targeted ketogenic diet (TKD): This diet allows you to feature carbs around workouts.

• High protein ketogenic diet: this is often almost like a typical ketogenic diet, but includes more protein. The ratio is usually 60% fat, 35% protein, and 5% carbs.

However, only the standard and high protein ketogenic diets are studied extensively. Cyclical or targeted ketogenic diets are more advanced methods and primarily used by bodybuilders or athletes.

The information in this article mostly applies to the quality ketogenic diet (SKD), although many of the same principles also apply to the opposite versions.

CHAPTER FOUR

What is ketosis?

Ketosis is a metabolic state during which your body uses fat for fuel rather than carbs.

It occurs once you significantly reduce your consumption of carbohydrates, limiting your body's supply of glucose (sugar), which is the main source of energy for the cells.

Following a ketogenic diet is the best way to enter ketosis. Generally, this involves limiting carb consumption to around 20 to 50 grams per day and filling abreast of fats, like meat, fish, eggs, nuts, and healthy oils

It's also important to moderate your protein consumption. this Or Add your own word:USEClick on original word (above) to restore.Click on any alternate word to replace.Click on Cross icon to close it."> this is often because protein can be converted into glucose if consumed in high amounts, which can slow your transition into ketosis).

Practicing intermittent fasting could also help you enter ketosis faster. There are many various sorts of intermittent fasting, but the foremost common method involves limiting food intake to around 8 hours per day and fasting for the remaining 16 hours

Blood, urine, and breath tests are available, which may help determine whether you've entered ketosis by measuring the quantity of ketones produced by your body.

Certain symptoms may additionally indicate that you've entered ketosis, including increased thirst, dry mouth, frequent urination, and decreased hunger or appetite

CHAPTER FIVE

Ketogenic Diets Can Assist You Lose Weight

A ketogenic diet is an effective way to lose weight and lower risk factors for disease

In fact, research shows that the ketogenic diet is also as effective for weight loss as a low fat diet What's more, the diet is so filling that you simply can reduce without counting calories or tracking your food

One review of 13 studies found that following a very low carb, ketogenic diet was slightly simpler for long-term weight loss than a low fat diet. people that followed the keto diet lost an average of two pounds (0.9 kg) quite the group that followed a low fat diet

What's more, it also led to reductions in diastolic blood pressure and triglyceride levels

Another study in 34 older adults found that those that followed a ketogenic diet for 8 weeks lost nearly five times the maximum amount total body fat as those that followed a low fat diet

The increased ketones, lower blood sugar levels, and improved insulin sensitivity can also play a key

CHAPTER SIX

Ketogenic Diets For Diabetes And Prediabetes

Diabetes is characterized by changes in metabolism, high blood sugar, and impaired insulin function

The ketogenic diet can help you lose excess fat, which is closely linked to type 2 diabetes, prediabetes, and metabolic syndrome

One older study found that the ketogenic diet improved insulin sensitivity by a whopping 75%

A small study in women with type 2 diabetes also found that following a ketogenic diet for 90 days significantly reduced levels of hemoglobin A1C, which is a measure of long-term blood sugar management Another study in 349 people with type 2 diabetes found that those that followed a ketogenic diet lost a mean of 26.2 pounds (11.9 kg) over a 2-year period. this is a very important benefit when considering the link between weight and type 2 diabetes

What's more, they also experienced improved blood sugar management, and also the use of certain blood glucose medications decreased among participants throughout the course of the study

Other health benefits of keto

The ketogenic diet actually originated as a tool for treating neurological diseases like epilepsy.

Studies have now shown that the diet can have benefits for a good form of different health conditions:

• Heart disease. The ketogenic diet can help improve risk factors like body fat, HDL (good) cholesterol levels, vital sign , and blood sugar

• Cancer. The diet is currently being explored as a further treatment for cancer, because it's going to help slow tumor growth.

• Alzheimer's disease. The keto diet may help reduce symptoms of Alzheimer's disease and slow its progression

• Epilepsy. Research has shown that the ketogenic diet can cause significant reductions in seizures in epileptic children

• Parkinson's disease. Although more research is required , one study found that the diet helped improve symptoms of Parkinson's disease

• Polycystic ovary syndrome. The ketogenic diet can help reduce insulin levels, which can play a key role in polycystic ovary syndrome

• Brain injuries. Some research suggests that the diet could improve outcomes of traumatic brain injuries

CHAPTER SEVEN

Foods To Avoid

Any food that's high in carbs should be limited.

Here's a list of foods that need to be reduced or eliminated on a ketogenic diet:

- sugary foods: soda, fruit juice, smoothies, cake, ice cream, candy, etc.

- grains or starches: wheat-based products, rice, pasta, cereal, etc.

- fruit: all fruit, except small portions of berries like strawberries

- beans or legumes: peas, kidney beans, lentils, chickpeas, etc.

- root vegetables and tubers: potatoes, sweet potatoes, carrots, parsnips, etc.

• low fat or diet products: low fat mayonnaise, salad dressings, and condiments

• some condiments or sauces: barbecue sauce, honey mustard, teriyaki sauce, ketchup, etc.

• unhealthy fats: processed vegetable oils, mayonnaise, etc.

• alcohol: beer, wine, liquor, mixed drinks

• sugar-free diet foods: sugar-free candies, syrups, puddings, sweeteners, desserts, etc.

CHAPTER EIGHT

Foods To Eat

You should base the majority of your meals around these foods:

• meat: red meat, steak, ham, sausage, bacon, chicken, and turkey

• fatty fish: salmon, trout, tuna, and mackerel

• eggs: pastured or omega-3 whole eggs

• butter and cream: grass-fed butter and cream

• cheese: unprocessed cheeses like cheddar, goat, cream, blue, or mozzarella

• nuts and seeds: almonds, walnuts, flaxseeds, pumpkin seeds, chia seeds, etc.

• healthy oils: extra virgin vegetable oil , coconut oil, and avocado oil

- avocados: whole avocados or freshly made guacamole
- low carb veggies: green veggies, tomatoes, onions, peppers, etc.
- condiments: salt, pepper, herbs, and spices

CHAPTER NINE

A Sample Keto Meal Plan For 1 Week

To help get you started, here's a sample ketogenic diet meal plan for one week:

Monday

• breakfast: veggie and egg muffins with tomatoes

• lunch: salad with vegetable oil , feta cheese, olives, and a side salad

• dinner: salmon with asparagus cooked in butter

Tuesday

• breakfast: egg, tomato, basil, and spinach omelet

• lunch: almond milk, peanut butter, spinach, cocoa powder, and stevia milkshake (more keto smoothies here) with a side of sliced strawberries

• dinner: cheese-shell tacos with salsa

Wednesday

• breakfast: nut milk chia pudding topped with coconut and blackberries

• lunch: avocado shrimp salad

• dinner: pork chops with Parmesan cheese, broccoli, and salad

Thursday

• breakfast: omelet with avocado, salsa, peppers, onion, and spices

• lunch: a couple of nuts and celery sticks with guacamole and salsa

• dinner: chicken full of pesto and cream cheese, and a side of grilled zucchini

Friday

• breakfast: sugar-free Greek, milk yogurt with peanut butter, cocoa powder, and berries

• lunch: ground beef lettuce wrap tacos with sliced bell peppers

• dinner: loaded cauliflower and mixed veggies

Saturday

• breakfast: cream cheese pancakes with blueberries and a side of grilled mushrooms

• lunch: Zucchini and beet “noodle” salad

• dinner: white fish cooked in coconut oil with kale and toasted pine nuts

Sunday

• breakfast: fried eggs with and mushrooms

• lunch: low carb sesame chicken and broccoli

• dinner: spaghetti squash Bolognese

CHAPTER TEN

Always try and rotate the vegetables and meat over the long term, as each type provides different nutrients and health benefits.

In case you get hungry between meals, here are some healthy, keto-approved snacks:

- fatty meat or fish
- cheese
- a few nuts or seeds
- keto sushi bites
- olives
- one or two hard-boiled or deviled eggs
- keto-friendly snack bars
- 90% dark chocolate

- full-fat Greek yogurt mixed with nut butter and cocoa powder
- bell peppers and guacamole
- strawberries and plain cottage cheese
- celery with salsa and guacamole
- beef jerky
- smaller portions of leftover meals
- fat bombs

CHAPTER ELEVEN

Keto Tips And Tricks

Although getting started on the ketogenic diet are often challenging, there are several tips and tricks that you simply can use to make it easier.

• Start by familiarizing yourself with food labels and checking the grams of fat, carbs, and fiber to see how your favorite foods can fit into your diet.

• Planning out your meals beforehand can also be beneficial and can assist you save additional time throughout the week.

• Many websites, food blogs, apps, and cookbooks also offer keto-friendly recipes and meal ideas that you simply can use to create your own custom menu.

• Alternatively, some meal delivery services even offer keto-friendly options for a fast and convenient way to enjoy keto meals at home.

• Look into healthy frozen keto meals when you're short on time

• When going to social gatherings or visiting family and friends, you will also want to think about bringing your own food, which can make it much

•

•Tips for eating out on a ketogenic diet

Many restaurant meals are often made keto-friendly.

Most restaurants offer some kind of meat or fish-based dish. Order this and replace any high carb food with extra vegetables.

Egg-based meals are also an excellent option, like an omelet or eggs and bacon.

Another favorite is bun-less burgers. you may also swap the fries for vegetables instead. Add extra avocado, cheese, bacon, or eggs.

At Mexican restaurants, you'll be able to enjoy any kind of meat with extra cheese, guacamole, salsa, and sour cream.

For dessert, ask for a mixed cheese board or berries with cream.

Side effects and how to reduce them

Although the ketogenic diet is usually safe for many healthy people, there could also be some initial side effects while your body adapts.

There's some anecdotal evidence of these effects often referred to as the keto flu .Based on reports from some on the eating plan, it's usually over within a couple of days.

Reported keto flu symptoms include diarrhea, constipation, and vomiting Other less common symptoms include:

- poor energy and mental function
- increased hunger
- sleep issues
- nausea
- digestive discomfort
- decreased exercise performance

To minimize this, you'll try a daily low carb diet for the first few weeks. this may teach your body to burn more fat before you completely eliminate carbs.

A ketogenic diet also can change the water and mineral balance of your body, so adding extra salt to your meals or taking mineral supplements may help. ask your doctor about your nutritional needs.

At least in the beginning, it's important to eat until you're full and avoid restricting calories too much. Usually, a ketogenic diet causes weight loss without intentional calorie restriction.

Risks Of The Keto Diet

Staying on the keto diet within the long term may have some negative effectsTrusted Source, including risks of the following:

- low protein in the blood
- extra fat in the liver
- kidney stones
- micronutrient deficiencies

A type of medication called sodium-glucose cotransporter 2 (SGLT2) inhibitors for type 2 diabetes can increase the danger for diabetic ketoacidosis, a dangerous condition that increases blood acidity. Anyone taking this medication should avoid the keto diet

More research is being done to determine the security of the keto diet in the long term. Keep your doctor informed of your eating decide to guide your choices.

Supplements for a ketogenic diet

Although no supplements are required, some can be useful.

• MCT oil. Added to drinks or yogurt, MCT oil provides energy and helps increase ketone levels. buy MCT oil online

www.ingramcontent.com/pod-product-compliance
Ingram Content Group UK Ltd.
Pitfield, Milton Keynes, MK11 3LW, UK
UKHW022009190726
13853UKWH00004B/1821

9 798423 396008